MEDIA
TECHNOLOGI

MW01519438

NOISE-INDUCED HEARING LOSS IN YOUTH CAUSED BY LEISURE NOISE

MEDIA AND COMMUNICATIONS – TECHNOLOGIES, POLICIES AND CHALLENGES

Videoconferencing: Technology, Impact and Applications
Adam C. Rayler (Editor)
2010. ISBN: 978-1-61668-285-9
2010. ISBN: 978-1-61668-407-5 (E-Book)

Tapping the Television White Space Spectrum: A Revolution in Public Airwave Use
Julie E. Hendriks (Editor)
2010. ISBN: 978-1-60692-956-8
2010. ISBN: 978-1-61728-439-7 (E-Book)

Digital Books: Competition and Commerce
Oliver A. Hagen (Editor)
2010. ISBN: 978-1-61728-299-7
2010. ISBN: 978-1-61728-450-2 (E-Book)

Information and Communication Technologies Policies and Practices
Almas Heshmati and Sun Peng (Editors)
2010. ISBN: 978-1-60876-671-0

Intelligibility Research and Communication Issues in Emergency Situations
Samuel A. Fletcher (Editor)
2010. ISBN: 978-1-61668-634-5
2010. ISBN: 978-1-61668-732-8 (E-Book)

Video Encryption Technology and Application
Zhengquan Xu and Jing Sun
2010. ISBN: 978-1-61668-331-3
2010. ISBN: 978-1-61668-734-2 (E-Book)

Reality Television – Merging the Global and the Local
Amir Hetsroni (Editor)
2010. ISBN: 978-1-61668-315-3

Noise-Induced Hearing Loss in Youth Caused by Leisure Noise
Hannah Keppler, B. Vinck and I. Dhooge
2010. ISBN: 978-1-61668-200-2
2010. ISBN: 978-1-61668-460-0 (E-Book)

Mediating Health: The Powerful Role of the Media
Deborah Begoray, Mimi Cimon and Joan Wharf Higgins
2010. ISBN: 978-1-61668-324-5
2010. ISBN: 978-1-61668-614-7 (E-Book)

Spectrum Issues for the New Communications Age
Caroline D. Underwood (Editor)
2010. ISBN: 978-1-61668-544-7
2010. ISBN: 978-1-61668-725-0 (E-Book)

The Newspaper Industry and Journalism in Transition
Rebecca E. Greene (Editor)
2010. ISBN: 978-1-61728-166-2
2010. ISBN: 978-1-61728-323-9 (E-Book)

MEDIA AND COMMUNICATIONS –
TECHNOLOGIES, POLICIES AND CHALLENGES

NOISE-INDUCED HEARING LOSS IN YOUTH CAUSED BY LEISURE NOISE

HANNAH KEPPLER

BART VINCK

AND

INGEBORG DHOO

Nova Science Publishers, Inc.
New York

For permission to use material from this book please contact us:
Telephone 631-231-7269; Fax 631-231-8175
Web Site: http://www.novapublishers.com

NOTICE TO THE READER
The Publisher has taken reasonable care in the preparation of this book, but makes no expressed or implied warranty of any kind and assumes no responsibility for any errors or omissions. No liability is assumed for incidental or consequential damages in connection with or arising out of information contained in this book. The Publisher shall not be liable for any special, consequential, or exemplary damages resulting, in whole or in part, from the readers' use of, or reliance upon, this material.

Independent verification should be sought for any data, advice or recommendations contained in this book. In addition, no responsibility is assumed by the publisher for any injury and/or damage to persons or property arising from any methods, products, instructions, ideas or otherwise contained in this publication.

This publication is designed to provide accurate and authoritative information with regard to the subject matter covered herein. It is sold with the clear understanding that the Publisher is not engaged in rendering legal or any other professional services. If legal or any other expert assistance is required, the services of a competent person should be sought. FROM A DECLARATION OF PARTICIPANTS JOINTLY ADOPTED BY A COMMITTEE OF THE AMERICAN BAR ASSOCIATION AND A COMMITTEE OF PUBLISHERS.

LIBRARY OF CONGRESS CATALOGING-IN-PUBLICATION DATA
Available upon request
ISBN: 978-1-61668-200-2

Published by Nova Science Publishers, Inc. ✦ New York

CONTENTS

PREFACE

The fact that excessive occupational noise exposure can lead to noise-induced hearing loss (NIHL) is well known. Besides this occupational noise exposure, non-occupational noise exposure is also a cause for concern, especially in young people. These leisure noise exposures include exposure to loud music or even participation in non-musical activities. The major sources of the former activities are attendance at discotheques, nightclubs and live concerts, and usage of personal music players. An increase in prevalence of NIHL in adolescents and young adults is assumed, especially in the mainstream media. Epidemiologic literature is, however, more equivocal. The purpose of this book is to give insight in the prevalence of NIHL caused by recreational noise exposure, and the sources of leisure noise. Research regarding temporary and permanent auditory effects caused by listening to personal music players and attending discotheques, nightclubs or live concerts is discussed. Shortcomings in the current literature are stressed, and proposals for additional research regarding the usefulness of several audiological tests to detect minimal cochlear damage after exposure to loud leisure noise on short- and long-term are suggested. Further, preventive strategies are discussed, and finally, the current legislation regarding leisure noise exposure is briefly reviewed.

H. Keppler, B. Vinck and I. Dhooge
Ghent, Belgium
October, 2009

Chapter 1

PATHOPHYSIOLOGY AND DIAGNOSIS OF NOISE-INDUCED HEARING LOSS

Sound perception is based on mechanical sound energy reaching the middle ear, inducing movement of the stapes footplate into the oval window, and producing pressure changes in the perilymph of the cochlea. The traveling wave of the basilar membrane (BM) deflects the stereocilia of the hair cells which stretches the tip links and forces them to open ionic channels on the stereocilia. The resulting potassium influx depolarizes the hair cells of the organ of Corti, and consequently releases neurotransmitters generating action potentials in the cochlear nerve by which neural afferent information is transferred to the brainstem. The motile activity of the outer hair cells (OHCs) [Brownell, 1990] amplifies the sound-induced micro-mechanical movement of the BM, especially at low-input levels. Thereby the input for the inner hair cells (IHCs) is enhanced. This non-linear active process, i.e. the cochlear amplifier, is responsible for the high sensitivity, sharp frequency selectivity and wide dynamic range of the human auditory system [Norton, 1992].

Excessive noise exposure can lead to metabolic and/or mechanical changes resulting in alterations of the structural elements of the Organ of Corti [Sliwinska-Kowalska and Jedlinska, 1998; Céranic, 2007; Talaska and Schacht, 2007]. Metabolic disturbances induce cell death through toxic reactions, while mechanical damage results in a direct physical loss of the integrity of hair cells and surroundings cells [Talaska and Schacht, 2007]. Morphological changes may include buckling of the pillar bodies, decreasing the height of the organ of Corti and thereby uncoupling the OHC stereocilia from the tectorial membrane [Nordmann et al, 2000]. This temporary uncoupling could affect hair cell stimulation, and is sufficient to explain temporary threshold shift (TTS). It is suggested that TTS and permanent threshold shift (PTS) arise from a fundamentally different mechanism [Nordmann et al, 2000], and that a PTS cannot be predicted form the initial TTS [Melnick, 1991] as it might depend on the recovery or repair processes within the cochlea [Nordmann et al, 2000]. Morphological correlates of PTS are focal losses of hair cells and adjacent afferent nerve fiber degeneration [Nordmann et al, 2000].

There are biochemical events that accompany morphological changes in the cochlea leading to degeneration of the sensory cells and eventually to degeneration of the spiral ganglion [Talaska and Schacht, 2007]. Prolonged noise exposure results in an accumulation of calcium, saturating the calcium-binding capacities of the OHCs [Heinrich and Feltens, 2006]. The disturbance of calcium homeostasis can result in an overload of calcium in the mitochondria, excitotoxic neural swelling, and reduction of cochlear blood flow. Thereby, reactive oxygen species (ROS) enzymes are activated and free radicals are generated [Henderson et al, 2006]. Although ROS formation is not limited to hair cells, but also occur in other structures such as supporting cells and the stria vascularis, the primary damage is concentrated on the OHCs [Sliwinska-Kowalska and Jedlinska, 1998; Lucertini et al, 2002; Sliwinska-Kowalska and Kotylo, 2007]. This might suggest that OHCs have a lower antioxidant capacity, and might therefore be more susceptible to ROS [Talaska and Schacht, 2007]. The co-existence of apoptosis and necrosis involved in OHC damage causes eventually cell death [Hu et al, 2002] and this induces disturbed physiological pathways in other cochlear cell types [Heinrich and Feltens, 2006]. Apoptosis is an active process that eliminates injured cells which could spread lesion to neighboring cells. The morphological correlate is nuclear condensation and fragmentation [Hu et al, 2002]. Necrosis, however, is a passive process associated with cell swelling resulting in cell rupture. Eventually, it results in damage to surrounding cells or inflammatory responses [Henderson et al, 2006]. However, necrosis is found to account for only a small portion of this damage, and apoptosis persists even several days after noise exposure [Hu et al, 2002]. Therefore, the clinical utility of delayed interventions must be further explored, as well as the role of antioxidant prevention of noise-induced hearing loss (NIHL) in humans [Le Prell et al, 2007].

Long periods of continuous or intermittent noise exposure can lead to a slowly developing chronic hearing loss, or NIHL. By analogy with NIHL, hearing loss caused by music is sometimes referred as music-induced hearing loss. Typically, noise is an unwanted, unpleasant acoustic signal [Hausler,

2004]. However, instead of the term music-induced hearing loss, the term NIHL is mainly used because noise is referred as an excessive acoustic signal possibly causing hearing damage, whether unwanted or not.

According to the Position Statement of the American College of Occupational and Environmental Medicine (ACOEM) on NIHL in 2002 (ACOEM, 2002), NIHL can be defined as a sensorineural, mostly bilateral symmetrical hearing loss initially presented in the frequency range 3 to 6 kHz. NIHL almost never progresses to a profound hearing loss, but the rate of hearing loss is greatest during the first 10 to 15 years of exposure and does not progress after cessation of noise exposure. However, it was postulated that hearing loss is only detected as soon as a considerable amount of hair cells is damaged [Daniel, 2007]. This suggests that there might be a period of latent damage making it impossible to distinguish audiometrically between subjects whether exposed to noise or not [LePage, 1998]. Moreover, the risk of hearing loss is influenced by the noise exposure level, duration, number of exposures and individual susceptibility [Mills and Going, 1982]. This individual susceptibility to noise seems to be related to the recovery processes within the cochlea after noise exposure.

Henderson (1993) states that there is a large variability in susceptibility to NIHL in demographic studies, as well as laboratory studies, which seemed to be caused by several factors. First, some of the variability could be explained by the interaction between noise exposure and other ototoxic agents exacerbating NIHL. Second, the role of auditory characteristics such as acoustic stapedial reflex, efferent system and subject's history of noise exposure could attribute to the variability of NIHL, and to a smaller extent, non-auditory characteristics such as gender, eye color and smoking [Henderson et al, 1993].

The diagnosis of NIHL is based on audiometric evaluation in combination with a history of noise exposure [Alberti, 1998]. Besides the loss of hearing sensitivity, concomitant tinnitus and impaired speech discrimination can be present. The sensitivity of pure-tone audiometry for the early detection of NIHL however has been questioned. The ACOEM has recommended additional research on NIHL, including in the area of early indicators of hearing loss such as otoacoustic emissions (OAEs) (ACOEM, 2002). OAEs are low-level sounds reflecting the non-linear active processes of the cochlea [Norton, 1992], which were discovered by Kemp in 1978 [Kemp, 1978]. It is a non-invasive, objective technique that does not require active participation of the subject. OAEs represent an indication of the integrity of the OHCs, but their presence does not exclude hearing impairment (e.g. retrocochlear hearing loss). However, OAEs depend highly on normal middle ear function [Probst et al 1991]. Nevertheless, OAE amplitude reduction may reflect OHC damage due to noise exposure [Sliwinska-Kowalska and Kotylo, 2007]. So, OAEs are a promising tool in the detection of sub-clinical OHC damage and pre-clinical hearing loss, overlooked by pure-tone audiometry. This has mainly been established in industrial or military settings [Hotz et al, 1993; Kowalska and Sulkowski, 1997; Hall and Lutman, 1999; Desai et al, 1999; Konopka et al, 2001; Attias et al, 2001; Lucertini et al, 2002; Céranic, 2007; Sliwinska-Kowalska and Kotylo, 2007]. Two types of OAEs, transiently evoked OAEs (TEOAEs) and distortion product OAEs (DPOAEs), are commonly used. In contrast to TEOAEs, DPOAEs have a more high-frequency response which makes them an ideal tool for detecting relatively high frequency-specific cochlear damage such as NIHL [Probst et al 1993]. However, some studies indicate that TEOAEs are more sensitive than DPOAEs in the detection of minimal cochlear alterations [Plinkert et al 1995; Lapsley-Miller et al 2004].

Chapter 2

PREVALENCE OF NOISE-INDUCED HEARING LOSS CAUSED BY LEISURE NOISE

In the mainstream media, an increase in prevalence of NIHL in adolescents and young adults attributable to recreational noise exposure is postulated. General statements regarding the prevalence of hearing loss in this generation are not uncommon ('more young people lose hearing', 'the deaf MP3 generation', etc.), but are usually based on possibilities or estimations. For example, in the United States, it was estimated that non-occupational noise exposure probably has a similar impact on the burden of adult hearing loss as occupational noise exposure which represents 5 to 10% of the burden [Dobie, 2008].

Two types of epidemiologic research can provide firm evidence; either cross-sectional studies or longitudinal data. However, there are methodological difficulties in the accurate estimation of the number of subjects exposed, and in obtaining a sample of young individuals with representative sound levels, patterns and duration of exposure [MRC Institute of Hearing Research, 1986]. Furthermore, the criteria used to define hearing impairment, and the used audiological techniques to measure slight deterioration in hearing, as well as numerous confounding factors in lifestyle regarding noise exposure (e.g. environmental noise) make the design of such research complicated. Finally, longitudinal studies require an adequate long-term planning, as well as identical methodological conditions.

Research regarding the prevalence of NIHL caused by leisure noise has revealed inconsistent results. There are some adequately performed studies that do not report an increase in prevalence of hearing loss caused by leisure noise.

First, the prevalence of hearing loss in 500 18-year-old males was 14%, which was comparable with the prevalence of hearing loss in the same age group in previous studies [Axelsson et al, 1994]. In 1998, the prevalence of hearing loss in 951 Swedish 18-year-old conscripts was estimated at 19.6% [Augustsson and Engstrand, 2006]. However, taking different techniques into account, the authors concluded that there is no increase in prevalence as compared with 30 years earlier [Persson et al, 1993].

Second, the Third National Health and Nutrition Examination Survey (NHANES III) [Niskar et al, 1998; Niskar et al, 2001], performed between 1988 and 1994, estimated the prevalence of a noise-induced threshold shift in children from 6 to 19 year old (n=5249). A noise-induced hearing threshold shift was defined as: (1) pure-tone thresholds at 0.5 and 1.0 kHz equal or better than 15 dB HL, (2) a difference of at least 15 dB between the poorest pure-tone threshold at 3.0, 4.0 or 6.0 kHz on the one hand and at 0.5 and 1.0 kHz on the other hand, and finally, (3) pure tone threshold at 8.0 kHz at least 10 dB better than the poorest threshold at 3.0, 4.0 and 6.0 kHz. It was stated that the prevalence of a noise-induced hearing threshold shift in at least one ear amounted to 12.5%, representing approximately 5.2 million children. In those children, the prevalence of noise-induced threshold shift was significantly higher in boys (14.8%) than in girls (10.1%). Further, it was observed that 12- to 19-year-old children had a significantly higher prevalence of noise-induced threshold shift (15.5%) than the 6- to 11-year-olds (8.5%). However, the median hearing thresholds of this oldest group of children can be compared with those of children aged 12 to 17 years from the Health Examination Survey of 1966 to 1970 [Holmes et al, 2004]. All median thresholds except at 1 kHz were better in children from the NHANES III, indicating better hearing conservation over the past 20 years. More importantly, the largest improvement was at frequencies 4 and 6 kHz, suggesting a decrease in hearing loss.

More recently, the prevalence of hearing loss was examined in US adults from 17 to 25 years entering an industrial workforce [Rabinowitz et al, 2006]. The criteria for an audiometric notch were defined identically as the noise-induced hearing threshold shifts by Niskar et al (2001). The prevalence of audiometric notches was 23.2% for the new-hires between 1985 and 1989, 17.2% between 1990 and 1994, 19.3% between 1995 and 1999, and 20.4% between 2000 and 2004. So, no increasing prevalence of audiometric notches, nor high frequency hearing loss (average hearing loss at 3, 4 and 6 kHz greater than 15 dB) was reported for hearing tests performed between 1985 and 2004.

There are, however, other studies reporting an increase in prevalence of hearing loss caused by leisure noise. Montgomery and Fujikawa (1992) evaluated hearing thresholds in almost 1500 students from second, eight and twelfth grade. The prevalence of hearing loss of second graders and eighth graders had increased compared to the prevalence of hearing loss ten years ago [Montgomery and Fujikawa, 1992]. However, the history of noise exposure was not investigated, and could therefore not been correlated with hearing loss. Similarly, a higher prevalence of impaired hearing, typically at high frequencies, was observed in children who started school in 1987 and 1997 than those who started in 1977 [Gissel et al, 2002]. In an interdisciplinary long-term study the effects of recreational noise exposure on hearing, and the correlation with psychosocial factors were yearly evaluated during a four-year period in adolescents (aged 14 to 17 years) [Biassoni et al, 2005]. During the third year, adolescents were divided into two subgroups based on hearing threshold shifts: small versus larger shifts. The ears of the adolescents in these subgroups were labeled as 'tough ears' or 'tender ears', respectively. The authors concluded that leisure activities associated with both subgroups could result in permanent hearing loss in adolescents with tender ears, but does not always cause hearing damage in tough ears.

Thus, the literature is so far not conclusive concerning the possible increase of NIHL caused by leisure noise. An extensive amount of literature investigated the relation between hearing loss and leisure noise exposure. Some found a high-frequency deterioration of hearing which was attributed to noise during leisure time [Litke, 1971; Lipscomb, 1972; Lees et al, 1985; Spaeth et al, 1993]. However, others found no or only slight correlation between hearing loss and leisure time noise exposure [Hanson and Fearn, 1975; Strauss et al, 1977; Axelsson et al, 1981a; Axelsson et al, 1981b; Carter et al, 1982; Carter et al, 1984; Bradley et al, 1987; Lindeman et al, 1987; Mercier and Hohmann, 2002]. A review by Zenner et al (1999), translated in Maassen et al (2001), indicated that the reason no correlation between music exposure and hearing loss was found, is based on methodological shortcomings such as averaging music exposure without dividing in subgroups with extreme exposure, testing non-suitable subgroups or no extreme groups with substantial (life time) exposure, and failing to obtain a control group without any music exposure. Furthermore, these authors stated:

> "We can conclude from the cited studies that the noise induced PTS, which has to be expected according to ISO 1999, has been sufficiently

demonstrated empirically, and that there is a considerable risk for ear damage resulting from electronically amplified music.",

and they further estimated that:

> "If the reported music listening habits of the 15 year olds are constant for 10 years, it can be expected that this will result in 10% of young Germans having an average hearing loss of 10 dB or more at 3 kHz. To this music-induce hearing loss, a further 10 dB hearing loss has to be added in 25 year olds due to age and therefore it can be expected that 10% of the 25 year olds have hearing thresholds above 20 dB at 3 kHz." [Zenner et al, 1999; Maassen et al, 2001].

Thus, it seems that the majority of properly designed research was not able to demonstrate a clear impact of leisure noise on auditory function. The most likely explanation for this lack of hearing deterioration could be that recreational noise exposure is insufficient to cause widespread hearing loss. It is plausible that the pattern of exposure to recreational noise is probably less frequent compared to occupational noise exposure, and attributes only for a small period in life probably between five and ten years [Hetu and Fortin, 1995; Axelsson and Prasher, 1999; Smith et al, 2000]. Moreover, individual behavior regarding use of hearing protectors might have changed [Rabinowitz et al, 2006] and/or there might be an alteration in noise exposure habits [Mostafapour et al, 1998] due to greater public awareness of the potential harmful effects of recreational noise exposure. However, it is also suggested that it is too soon to detect permanent effects of recent advances in technology [Morata, 2007], such as MP3 players. Finally, pure-tone audiometry is possibly not the most sensitive technique to detect subtle cochlear changes, and other measures – high-frequency audiometry, high-definition audiometry and OAEs – might reveal subclinical cochlear damage. For example, significant weakening of TEOAEs was found in adolescents more exposed to amplified music than the less exposed adolescents [Mansfield et al, 1999].

Besides hearing loss, there is a high prevalence of tinnitus reported in individuals with occupational NIHL [Axelsson and Prasher, 2000]. While there seems to be an increased awareness of noise exposure in occupational settings, it is plausible that the prevalence of tinnitus due to recreational noise exposure is on the rise. In subjects reporting tinnitus, the level of social noise exposure determines the audiological characteristics as measured with pure-tone audiometry, speech-in-noise test, and otoacoustic emissions [Davis et al, 1998]. Also, it was found that 8.7% of 1285 Swedish participants between 13 and 19 years reported tinnitus, and 17.1% reported noise sensitivity [Widen and Erlandsson, 2004]. Both symptoms were more common in older than younger adolescents which could be explained by the longer period of leisure noise exposure. Thus, subjective audiological symptoms including tinnitus and hypersensitivity to sound should be considered in the evaluation of temporary or permanent thresholds shifts because it might indicate subtle cochlear changes [Schmuziger et al, 2006]. Tinnitus is also found to be a more suffering symptom than hearing loss [Metternich and Brusis, 1999; Axelsson and Prasher, 1999]. Therefore, more research is needed to estimate the prevalence of non-occupational noise-induced permanent tinnitus.

In summary, there is a large amount of research concerning the impact of leisure noise exposure on hearing, especially during music-related activities. However, the majority of these studies are characterized with poor methodology which leads to inconsistent results regarding a correlation between these aforementioned activities and hearing damage, as well as an assumed increase in prevalence of hearing loss caused by these activities. Nevertheless, in our opinion, as long as firm evidence based on adequately executed research is lacking, caution is necessary. As such, more research is urgently needed to gain more insight.

Chapter 3

LEISURE NOISE ACTIVITIES

Generally, recreational noise exposure can be categorized into exposure to loud music or participation in non-musical activities. The major sources of music-related leisure noise are: (1) using personal music players (PMPs), (2) attendance at nightclubs or discotheques, (3) attendance at live concerts, (4) listening to home stereo/ radio's, and (5) playing a musical instrument, playing in a band or an orchestra [MRC Institute of Hearing Research, 1986; Clark, 1991; Meyer-Bisch, 1996; Jokitulppo et al, 1997; Mansfield et al, 1999; Smith et al, 2000; Jokitulppo and Bjork, 2002; Jokitulppo et al, 2006]. Loud music listening is possible in almost every surroundings; associated with activities at home, while driving or traveling by bike, bus, train or underground [Rice et al, 1987a; Wong et al, 1990].

Smith et al (2000) studied the prevalence and type of social noise in England in an age group between 18 to 25 years. It was found that the prevalence of recreational noise in the UK since the early 1980s has tripled from 6.7% to 18.8%, whereas occupational noise was decreased from 8.9% to 3.5%. About 11% received significant noise exposure from nightclubs, 3% from Hi-fis, 2% from PMPs, and 0.6% from attendance at live concerts. Significant noise exposure was defined as a situation in which raised voices between two normal hearing people four feet apart holding an conversation are needed [Smith et al, 2000]. Jokitulppo and Björk (2002) investigated the noisy leisure-time of Finnish adults (25-58 years) and found that 58% listened to a home stereo/radio, 34% went to nightclubs/pubs, 9% used a portable stereo player, 7% attended at live concerts, and only a small amount played a musical instrument (7%), in a band (1%) or orchestra (1%) [Jokitulppo and Bjork, 2002]. In Argentina, participation of adolescents in musical recreational activities was found highest for attendance at discotheques, followed consecutively by attendance at live concerts, usage of PMPs and playing musical instruments [Serra et al, 2005].

Thus, the contribution of PMPs to the total social noise exposure seems to be less than the attendance of discotheques or nightclubs. Recently however, it was found that more than 90% of 1016 American students listened to some type of personal music system through earphones [Torre, 2008]. It seems plausible that the technical evolution since the introduction of the Sony Walkman to the MPEG layer-3 (MP3) players has contributed to the current popularity of PMPs. There has been a miniaturization of the devices, an improvement of the storage and battery capacity, and online availability of music and podcasts. Thus, it is not known if findings from other PMPs – personal cassette players (PCPs) or Compact Disc players (CD players) - apply directly to MP3 player use [Vogel et al, 2007]. For example, there was a 5 dB increase in averaged levels between CD players and MP3 players using the same measurement technique [Keith et al, 2008]. Therefore, the effects of PMPs and especially MP3 players on the auditory system of young people is a cause for concern. This concern is based on the close coupling of headphones to the tympanic membrane, the ability of such devices to generate high maximum output levels, and uncertainties regarding listening habits.

Besides these music-related leisure noise sources, there are other sources of leisure noise such as attending or participating in sport events and motor sport events, watching movies or going to the theatre, using home tools, shooting firearms, use of fireworks, and other noisy toys. Participation in non-musical activities is, however, less common than in musical activities [Biassoni et al, 2005], and the highest participation in non-musical activities is watching movies or going to the theatre (26%), and using home tools indoors (19%) [Jokitulppo and Bjork, 2002].

1. PERSONAL MUSIC PLAYERS

1.1. Listening Habits

There is a large variation in listening habits of adolescents using PMPs, between studies, as well as within studies. This variation is seen in duration of use (years), listening time (hours per week) and listening levels. It can largely be explained by the studied population; either no representative population was studied [e.g. Williams, 2005], or there were differences in sociodemographic characteristics in subjects between studies. Moreover, differences in questions regarding using PMPs explain the inconsistencies between studies. For example, the listening time is sometimes referred to as listening during one single session [Zogby, 2006], or for a full day [Torre, 2008]. Thereby, adequate comparisons in listening habits between studies are difficult. With consideration of these shortcomings, there are, however, some tendencies regarding listening habits with respect of gender and age.

First, females spend less time listening to PMPs [Catalano and Levin, 1985; Rice et al, 1987a; Meyer-Bisch, 1996; Torre, 2008], and prefer to listen at less intensive output levels [Catalano and Levin, 1985; Smith et al, 2000; Williams, 2005; Torre, 2008].

Catalano and Levin (1985) found that females listened on average 8.04 hours per week, whereas the average for males was 13.97 hours per week [Catalano and Levin, 1985]. Rice et al (1987a) reported that males listen on average about one hour per week more to their PCPs than females [Rice et al, 1987a]. Moreover, there was a higher percentage of females only occasionally listening to PCPs (17.3%) than males (10.9%) [Meyer-Bisch, 1996]. Further, it was found that 25.2% of the females used a PCP for at least two hours per week, whereas in males this was 37.6%. Recently, Torre (2008) reported that 11.2% more females listen to PMPs less than one hour per day. In contrast, 5.4% more males listened between one and three hours, 4.6% more males between three and five hours, and finally, 1.2% more males listened longer than five hours per day as compared to the females [Torre, 2008].

On average, males set their PCP 7.5 dB higher than females [Smith et al, 2000]. The mean eight hour, A-weighted equivalent continuous noise level was 75.3 dB for the females, and 80.6 dB for the males [Williams, 2005]. Also, medium volume setting of PMPs was preferred for most women, whereas men were more likely to listen at a very loud listening level [Torre, 2008].

Second, listening habits tend to changes during lifetime [Fearn and Hanson, 1984; West and Evans, 1990; Smith et al, 2000; Meyer-Bisch, 1996; Zogby, 2006; Zenner et al, 1999; Maassen et al, 2001].

The percentage of young people listening through headphones increased from 10%, 12% and 35% for the age groups 9 to 12 years, 13 to 16 years and 18 to 25 years, respectively [Fearn and Hanson, 1984]. In contrast, the use of PMPs decreased from 67% in younger (15-16 years) to 39% in older (19-23 years) exposed adolescents [West and Evans, 1990]. Moreover, the most frequent use of PCP was reported to range between 13 and 19 years [Smith et al, 2000], and Meyer-Bisch (1996) mentioned less often usage of PCPs after the age of 28 [Meyer-Bisch, 1996]. The percentage of high school (14-18 years) students using an Apple iPod or another brand of MP3 player was three times as high than for adults (18-+70 years), indicating that usage declines with increasing age [Zogby, 2006].

Median PMP listening duration increased from 16 years, with a median of approximately one hour 20 minutes at the age of 19 years [Zenner et al, 1999; Maassen et al, 2001]. In 2006, the length of a typical session of PMP usage was reported to range between one and four hours for a larger amount of adults, and between 30 minutes and one hour for students [Zogby, 2006].

Median listening levels were above 90 dBA between the ages of 13 and 16 years, reaching a median level of almost 100 dBA at 14 years [Zenner et al, 1999; Maassen et al, 2001]. Moreover, the typical volume setting for a student listening to a PMP was more often loud, somewhat loud or very loud, whereas adults listen to PMPs more at medium, somewhat low, low or very low volume settings [Zogby, 2006].

Besides gender and age differences in the output level of PMPs, the preferred listening levels of these devices depend on several other factors, such as the presence of background noise, the type of music, the earphone style, and the type of personal music device.

First, it was found that the presence of background noise increases the preferred listening levels. The results depend on whether the measurements were performed in laboratory or field conditions. For example, Rice et al (1987b) found a signal-to-noise ratio (SNR) of approximately 5 dB in laboratory conditions, whereas in the field study no correlation was seen of listening levels with background traffic noise [Rice et al, 1987b]. In contrast, the preferred listening levels in laboratory conditions had on average a SNR of 12 dB, and in the field condition 17 dB [Airo et al, 1996]. Recently, the mean SNR in 55 subjects ranging in age from 15 to 48 years was about 13 dB measured at public areas [Williams, 2005]. Finally, the increase in preferred listening levels of an MP3 player in 38 subjects from 20 to 36 years was on average 9.4 dB higher for street noise and 7.7 dB higher for multi-talker babble, as compared to the quiet condition [Hodgetts et al, 2007]. Thus, it is important to evaluate the preferred listening levels of PMPs in the presence of background levels as these potentially result in a higher risk of hearing-related symptoms. Furthermore, increasing the listening levels might pose users at risk by decreasing their ability to hear warning signals. As such, adolescents should be advised to adjust the volume control of PMPs in quiet conditions.

Second, the preferred listening levels might be dependent on the type of music. One study evaluated the preferred listening levels for four music samples and found a difference of 10 dB between the quietest and loudest average listening levels in 14 subjects (16-26 years) [Airo et al, 1996]. Maximum output levels for different types of music were investigated by Turunen-Rise et al (1991) and more extensively by Fligor and Cox (2004). In the former study, sound pressure levels ranged from 100 to 108 dBA for pop music, 103 dBA for light classical music, and 98 dBA for classical music [Turunen-Rise et al, 1991]. Fligor and Cox (2004) measured maximum output levels of CD players for eight different styles of music relative to white noise. Country, rock and adult contemporary music samples were similar to the output levels measured with white noise. However, the output levels of the other music samples were overestimated by the white noise output levels. These overestimations were 2.5 dB, 3.9 dB, 4.9 dB, 5.6 dB and 12 dB for rap/ RandB, pop music, classical music, dance music and jazz, respectively. Moreover, the temporal pattern of these genres were evaluated. It was noticed that the highest peak SPLs were seen during the 10-sec rock and pop music sample, whereas the highest continuous 10-sec average SPL was during the rock sample. Further, dance music revealed the highest number of peaks in the 10-sec sample within 3 dB of the highest peak, and the temporal pattern of the jazz music sample was least pronounced. The number of transients during the 10-sec dance music sample ranged from 28 to 60 depending on the combination of CD player and headphone [Fligor and Cox, 2004].

Third, the earphone style determines the preferred listening levels of PMPs. Preferred listening levels were on average 1.3 dB higher for the supra-aural earphones than with semi-aural earphones [Airo et al, 1996]. Further, significant lower preferred listening levels were chosen for the over-the-ear headphone as compared to earbuds [Hodgetts et al, 2007]. This difference was 2.6 dB in quiet, 4.3 dB in presence of street noise and 3.8 dB with multi-talker babble. Also, it was reported that earbuds produce significant higher maximum output levels than supra-aural headphones, up to 7 dB [Fligor and Cox 2004]. MacLean et al (1992) found a 6.2 dB higher output level for the earbuds than for the supra-aural headphones. The differences might be explained by the physical coupling of the headphones, as well as their differences in operating characteristics [MacLean et al, 1992]. Finally, output levels of a tight fit of earbuds and supra-aural headphones were on average 16 dB higher than those of a loose fitting [Keith et al, 2008]. Thus, the coupling of the ear- and headphone, as well as the geometry of the ear defines the noise exposure using PMPs.

1.2. Short- and Long-Term Auditory Effects

Generally, temporary reduction in hearing sensitivity may be the result of listening to high output levels of PMPs during a short period (hours), while permanent hearing deterioration may be caused by listening to PMPs during a much longer period (years), even at lower listening levels. As mentioned previously, the exact relationship between TTS and PTS is uncertain. However, it is assumed that in the long term temporary hearing shifts may result in permanent hearing reduction.

Short-term effects of listening to PMPs were investigated measuring hearing thresholds, and recently, also by OAEs before and after a listening session. Lee et al (1985) found significant TTSs of 10 dB in 6 of the 16 subjects, as well as a TTS of approximately 30 dB in one subject after listening to three-hour during music with output levels ranging from 80 to 104 dB SPL [Lee et al, 1985]. Turunen-Rise et al (1991) described median TTSs of less than 12 dB after one hour listening to two types of pop music at a preset listening level between 85 and 95 dBA in six subjects [Turunen-Rise et al, 1991]. Hellström (1991) evaluated TTSs after exposure to one hour modern music via PCP at loud, but comfortable volume. The mean listening levels ranged from 91 to 97 dBA with mean TTS from 4.01 to 5.74 dB [Hellstrom, 1991]. Loth et al (1992) found an average TTS of 5 dB in 12 subjects after one-hour at preferred equivalent levels between 89 and 94 dBA [Loth et al, 1992]. Pugsley et al (1993) reported no significant larger deterioration in hearing after listening to a PMP during one hour in 30 subjects than in the control group of 15 subjects [Pugsley et al, 1993]. Hellström et al (1998) exposed 21 subjects to music via PCP at a loud, but comfortable level. Subjects were divided in three groups depending on their listening pattern. The average equivalent listening levels were 91.4 dBA, 91.9 dBA and 97.1 dBA with mean TTSs 15.7 dB, 4.5 dB and 4.0 dB, respectively [Hellstrom et al, 1998]. Recently, Bhagat and Davis (2008) measured hearing thresholds, DPOAEs and synchronized SOAEs (SSOAEs) in 20 subjects after listening to music during 30 minutes at a preset listening level. There were no significant differences in hearing thresholds before and after music exposure. There were, however, significant reductions in DPOAE half-octave band levels centered from 1.4 to 6.0 kHz, but variable shifts in frequency and level of SSOAEs [Bhagat and Davis, 2008].

From these TTS studies, we may be conclude that there are only slight, if any, reductions in hearing thresholds after listening to PMPs, but changes in OAEs might be early warning signs of the harmful effects of high levels of music exposure. There are however some shortcomings, as well as considerable variability in literature regarding temporary hearing damage after listening to PMPs. First, there is only one study [Pugsley et al, 1993] which included a control group to evaluate the threshold changes in a experimental group based on the test-retest reliability of hearing thresholds in a control group. Second, Lee et al (1985) considered thresholds shifts of at least 10 dB to be significant while others only reported the mean or median TTS [Hellstrom, 1991; Turunen-Rise et al, 1991; Hellstrom et al, 1998]. Third, there are methodological differences in music exposure, as well as in the determination of output levels. The music exposure ranged from one hour to three hours with different genres of music: with rock/fusion music [Lee et al, 1985], pop music [Turunen-Rise et al, 1991], contemporary music [Pugsley et al, 1993] or the favorite music cassette of the subjects [Hellstrom, 1991; Hellstrom et al, 1998]. Mainly, user-preferred listening levels were used with either standard headphones [Hellstrom, 1991; Turunen-Rise et al, 1991; Hellstrom et al, 1998] or user-preferred headphones [Lee et al, 1985]. However, one study [Pugsley et al, 1993] did not perform output measures to correlate with the results from the hearing test. The output levels were measured on an artificial ear with coupler [Lee et al, 1985], on KEMAR [Turunen-Rise et al, 1991], or via a miniature microphone in the external ear canal [Hellstrom, 1991; Hellstrom et al, 1998].

There are also several studies investigating the permanent auditory effects caused by long-term listening to PMPs. Wong et al (1990) found no differences in mean hearing thresholds between 78 young PCP users and 25 non-users [Wong et al, 1990]. However, the half-octave frequencies 3.0 and 6.0 kHz were not reported. Meyer-Bisch (1996) compared high definition audiometry in three groups. There were significant poorer hearing thresholds in the most exposed PCP group (n=54, >7hrs/wk) compared to the controls (n=358). No significant differences were seen between the less exposed PCP group (n=195, 2-7 hrs/wk) and the control group. There was also twice more subjective auditory suffering - presence of tinnitus and/or hearing fatigue - in the total PCP group than in the controls [Meyer-Bisch, 1996]. LePage and Murray (1998) noticed a decline in click-evoked OAEs significantly proportional with increasing PCP listening time from less than one hour to more than six hours per week [LePage and Murray, 1998]. Mostafapour et al (1998) evaluated hearing thresholds, speech reception threshold and speech discrimination in 50 subjects with estimated lifetime exposure of PMPs low, medium or high. No significant differences between the three groups were found [Mostafapour et al, 1998]. Peng et al (2007) found significant differences in hearing thresholds at conventional and extended high-frequencies between 120 PMP users and 30 controls, but no significant differences between the three subgroups of PMP use (one to three years, three to five years, longer than five years) were seen. Moreover, the hearing thresholds at extended high-frequencies of normal-hearing subjects at conventional frequencies were significantly higher than those of the control group. Therefore, the authors concluded that long-term use of PMPs could induce NIHL, and extended high-frequency audiometry is more sensitive than audiometry at conventional frequencies [Peng et al, 2007]. Montoya et al (2008) found a reduction of TEOAE and DPOAE incidence and amplitudes, as well as an increase in DPOAE thresholds with longer duration of listening to PMPs in years, and for more hours per week [Montoya et al, 2008].

The result of the aforementioned studies might indicate that with more extensive use of PMPs, hearing deteriorates. However, several shortcomings in these studies can be pointed out. First, in some studies [LePage and Murray, 1998; Peng et al, 2007], there was no consideration of other sources of leisure noise. So, it is impossible to distinguish hearing damage caused by PMPs from deterioration caused by several confounding sources of leisure noise. Second, mostly either the duration of use in years [Peng et al, 2007], or the use per week [Meyer-Bisch, 1996; LePage and Murray, 1998] of PMPs was investigated. In our opinion, the lifetime noise exposure from PMPs must be evaluated encompassing both parameters. Third, in some studies, subjects were not representative for the population [Wong et al, 1990; Mostafapour et al, 1998]. It is possible that with a more representative group, more extreme listening habits appear. Finally, the mentioned listening habits are based on a retrospective estimation by the subjects which could lead to errors in the quantification of PMP usage.

Previously, risk assessments were established, and ranged from 0.065 to 30% [Catalano and Levin, 1985; MRC Institute of Hearing Research, 1986; Rice et al, 1987a; Clark, 1991; Ising et al, 1994; Ising et al, 1995; Passchier-Vermeer, 1999; Williams, 2005]. Moreover, PMPs are supplementary sound sources and might accumulate with other noise exposure [Meyer-Bisch, 1996]. The variability in risk assessment could be explained by the definition for NIHL and the damage-risk criteria for hearing loss, which are directly adopted from occupational settings. According to some authors, extrapolation of occupational risk criteria to leisure noise exposures is not justified because of the differences in spectral and temporal pattern between industrial noise and music [Turunen-Rise et al 1991; Mostafapour et al 1998; Metternich and Brusis, 1999; Smith et al 2000; Fligor and Cox 2004]. Amplified music

emphasizes low-frequencies, and is characterized with transients superimposed on a relatively steady-state signal [Peng et al, 2007]. As such, it can be assumed that A-weighted sound levels underestimate the low-frequency contribution, and C-weighted sound levels could be proposed. However, industrial criteria are usually expressed in dBA. Moreover, it was also found that aversive sounds – noise or disliked music - induced larger TTSs than enjoyable sounds [Lindgren and Axelsson, 1983; Swanson et al, 1987]. Nevertheless, the regulation for occupational noise exposure is based on the exposure level and duration of noise exposure which also determines leisure noise exposure and there are currently no criteria available for this latter source. Thus, the criteria adopted from occupational noise exposure can be applied to evaluate the impact of leisure noise, although this must be done with caution. Therefore, users should be warned for the gradual and insidious development of hearing loss associated with long-term listening to PMPs at high intensity levels [Smith et al, 2000].

2. ATTENDANCE AT DISCOTHEQUES, NIGHTCLUBS OR LIVE CONCERTS

2.1. Attendance Habits

Generally, it is assumed that discotheques or nightclubs have a larger impact on young people's hearing than concerts. The noise exposure in the latter can be louder, but are attended less frequently and leading to less overall noise immission [Smith et al, 2000; Serra et al, 2005]. In 700 adolescents ranging in age from 16 to 25 years, attending discotheques regularly was found to be 79%, whereas attendance at pop and rock concerts and techno parties was 53% and 36% respectively [Mercier and Hohmann, 2002]. The average hours per week in 1323 adolescents (age range 28-58 years) was 4.4 for nightclubs/ pubs and 2.4 for concerts [Jokitulppo et al, 2006]. An average of 6.2 hours per week was determined for discotheque attendance [Zenner et al, 1999; Maassen et al, 2001].

Some tendencies regarding gender and age differences can be found in discotheque, nightclubs or concert attendance. First, more males (91%) attended nightclubs than females (84%) which was investigated in 494 university students [Meecham and Hume, 2001]. Meyer-Bisch (1996) also found more occasionally discotheque attendance in females, and more frequent attendance (at least twice a month) by males. Further, a higher proportion of males regularly (once a month) or intensively (twice a month) attended concerts [Meyer-Bisch, 1996]. Second, attending discotheques and concerts was reported more often in older exposed (19-23 years) than younger exposed (15-16 years) adolescents [West and Evans, 1990]. Moreover, the highest proportion of attendance was at 21-22 years, and rare after 28 years [Meyer-Bisch, 1996]. It was reported that the highest median visits per month was at the age of 17-18 years, with a decreasing trend from 22 years [Zenner et al, 1999; Maassen et al, 2001]. However, the more extreme noise exposure habits indicate that visits of more than twice a month was exceeded at the age of 13 years, with the highest 10% value of approximately seven visits a month at 19 years.

The mean of sound levels, measured in discotheques and rock concerts was 103.4 dBA [Clark, 1991]. Smith et al (2000) reported sound levels in nightclubs and discotheques ranging from 85 to 105 dBA with a mean of 101 dBA [Smith et al, 2000]. Another study found sound levels in nightclubs in the range of 97 to 106 dBA [Meecham and Hume, 2001]. Factors influencing these sound levels are: measurement position, time in the evening, variations between clubs, as well as between evenings in the same club [Ising, 1994; Smith et al, 2000; Meecham and Hume, 2001]. Recently, average sound levels for concerts ranged from 95 to 102 dBA for pop concerts, 97 to 103 dBA for heavy metal concerts, and 96 to 107 dBA for rock concerts with maximum sound levels 126, 113 and 118 dBA, respectively [Opperman et al, 2006]. So, it is clearly a misconception that some music genres, especially rock and heavy metal concerts, are louder than pop concerts.

As in listening habits of PMPs, it is difficult to establish general attendance habits in a representative sample of adolescents. Moreover, there are only few studies addressing the sound levels with respect of the influencing parameters.

2.2. Short- and Long-Term Effects

Clark (1991) reported that research in the seventies and eighties regarding temporary auditory effects indicates moderate TTS up to 30 dB recovering within hours to days after noise exposure [Clark, 1991]. For example, Axelsson and Lindgren (1978) found mean TTSs at 4 kHz of approximately 12 dB in listeners, and 10 dB in pop musicians. TTSs amounted up to 45 dB HL [Axelsson and Lindgren, 1978]. More recently, in a small population (n=22)

TTSs after rock concerts were found to be 10.9, 9.8 and 20.9 dB depending on the position in the arena with respective L_{Aeq} of 89.29, 99.6 and 101.3 dBA [Yassi et al, 1993]. Peak levels were almost 140 dBA which is assumed to cause irreversible acoustic trauma due to impulse noise. Sixty percent of the subjects assessed the sound levels as too loud or intolerable. However, only slightly more than half the subjects were aware of their TTSs which is a cause for concern and emphasizes the insidious nature of NIHL. The average TTS after attending discotheques increased from 6.2 dB to 10.01 dB with increasing attendance from one to two hours [Liebel et al, 1996]. Significant effects on TEOAE reproducibility and amplitudes were also found, but not on DPOAEs. Opperman et al (2006) found that largest mean hearing shifts were located at 3 and 4 kHz. Significant hearing shifts, according to OSHA and ASHA criteria, were present in 64% of the subjects wearing no earplugs, whereas in 27% wearing earplugs. This might be explained by the fact that the real-world attenuation of hearing protection devices is less than theoretically established mainly by the fitting of the earplugs into ear canal [Opperman et al, 2006]. Therefore, it is important to instruct adolescents correctly wearing earplugs.

The permanent auditory effects of concert and discotheque attendance in adolescents can be considered more dangerous than the use of PMPs [Meyer-Bisch, 1996; Mercier and Hohmann, 2002; Biassoni et al, 2005]. However, only few studies evaluated the long-term auditory effects of attending discotheques, nightclubs or concerts. Meyer-Bisch (1996) noticed a significant reduction in hearing thresholds, especially at 4 kHz, in the concert group as compared to the control group which never or only occasionally used a PMP and went only rarely to concerts or discotheques [Meyer-Bisch, 1996]. No significant differences in hearing thresholds between the discotheque attendees and control group could be established. However, there was three times more auditory suffering in the discotheque group than the controls, whereas in the concert group this was four times higher than in the control group. Meecham and Hume (2001) reported no significant association between attendance of nightclubs and occurrence of post exposure tinnitus, but they indicate that attendance increased the risk of and reduced recovery from tinnitus after noise exposure [Meecham and Hume, 2001].

3. CONCLUSION

It can be concluded that there is a large variation in listening and attendance habits of the most popular music-related leisure noise activities. Gender and age differences are two major sociodemographic factors partially explaining the variation in habits. More research is needed to extensively evaluate the type of leisure noise activities, as well as listening or attendance habits in a representative sample of adolescents.

TTS studies indicate that there are only slight reductions in hearing thresholds after listening to PMPs, but more damage seems to be present after attending discotheques, nightclubs or live concerts. However, more sensitive methods to evaluate minimal cochlear changes should be incorporated in future TTS studies with consideration of the mentioned shortcomings of the existing studies.

Furthermore, PTS studies indicate that visiting discotheques, nightclubs or concerts poses more risk to hearing than listening to PMPs. The measured sound pressures levels indicate theoretically that frequently attending these activities might cause hearing loss. As previously mentioned however, a clear association between hearing loss and attendance of these activities has not been proven yet, and more research is needed addressing hearing loss in young people with more extensive listening habits for multiple sources of leisure noise.

Chapter 4

PREVENTION OF NOISE-INDUCED HEARING LOSS CAUSED BY LEISURE NOISE

It is currently inconceivable that several parties such as weddings would take place without music exposure. However, it is remarkable that young people tend to listen to music in almost every environment, individually using their PMPs, as in groups in discotheques, nightclubs, concerts festivals etc. Plath (1998) describes this phenomenon as the fear of silence, as well as the reduction of unwanted background noise by listening to music [Plath, 1998a; Plath, 1998b]. However, adolescents extent this behavior to excessive music-listening in which music has to be felt, consistent with exuberant behavior [Clark, 1991]. Zenner et al (1999) and Maassen et al (2001) mentioned that such behavior compensates for the frustration and problems experienced by adolescents [Zenner et al, 1999; Maassen et al, 2001]. Florentine et al (1998) stated that music-listening behavior is sometimes associated with dependency-like disorders [Florentine et al, 1998], and recently, it was found that there was a correlation between general risk behavior such as smoking, drinking and leaving school on the one hand, and risk behavior regarding loud music on the other hand [Bohlin and Erlandsson, 2007].

Hetu and Fortin (1995) analyzed the temporal and spectral features of discotheque music, especially house music. It was postulated that the pulsating character of house music influences cardiac activity, and thus the general level of arousal. Moreover, low-frequency emphasizing maximizes beat perception, mid-frequency reduction prevents annoyance by permitting communication, and high-frequency enhancement allows perception of high-pitched sounds to stress the beat. Furthermore, these authors described the phenomenology of music-listening explaining the possessing of music. First, penetration of the music environment is limited due to the high sound pressure levels, as well as uninterrupted nature of discotheque or nightclub music (confinement). Second, listeners are enclosed in a musical field shared by other listeners (immersion). Third, music is heard without any focus or attention needed; communication is hardly impossible (passive hearing). Finally, the music and the light show are responsible for auditory, vestibular and proprioceptive sensations (excitement) [Hetu and Fortin, 1995].

The opposite of such excessive social lifestyle is presented when adolescents experience a hearing loss which affects their quality of life [Arlinger, 2003]. The handicap of NIHL in adolescents has an impact on the individual in interactions, but also in their broader communications with family and friends, as well as on the society. Their educational achievement is hampered, and eventually also their employability. In Argentina, pre-employment medical examination is failed in a high percentage of young people because of hearing loss [Serra et al, 2005]. Therefore, it is important to prevent NIHL, in occupational settings, but also during leisure activities.

Preventive strategies should incorporate a two-layered approach. First, by educating the adolescents and second, by protective measures such as legislation. It was reported that not only adolescents, but several other parties are involved in the prevention of NIHL. To prevent NIHL caused by discotheque attendance, the authorities, discotheque owners and decorators, as well as disc-jockeys are possible responsible [Vogel et al, 2009a]. Preventing NIHL due to PMP-listening, manufacturers of earphones and MP3 players, authorities, music industry, parents, media and community centers are potentially involved [Vogel et al, 2009b].

Improving the awareness and knowledge regarding the problems associated with excessive loud music-listening, consequences and preventive measures should be aimed for. Chung et al (2005) conducted a web-based survey, and found that only 8% of the 3310 respondents indicate hearing loss as a 'very big problem' [Chung et al, 2005]. Among the seven health concerns – hearing loss, sexually transmitted diseases, alcohol or drug abuse, depression, smoking, nutrition and weight issues and acne – hearing loss was perceived as the least 'very big problem'. Further, others reported that knowledge regarding the irreversibility of NIHL was limited [Weichbold and Zorowka, 2002; Shah et al, 2009]. Others have found a greater awareness of the risks in their population [Crandell et al, 2004; Rawool and Colligon-Wayne, 2008]. However, since there is still a great deal of unawareness, or al lot of misconceptions regarding to NIHL caused by leisure noise, information is necessary. Hearing education campaigns improve knowledge and awareness of NIHL, and improve motivation to protect the hearing [Becher et al, 1996]. However, it was found that the behavior of adolescents did not change: the frequency of discotheque attendance after a hearing education campaign even increased, the average duration of discotheque attendance, the use of hearing protection and their listening behavior using headphones was not influenced by the campaign [Weichbold and Zorowka, 2002; Weichbold and Zorowka, 2003; Weichbold and Zorowka, 2007]. Only the use of regeneration breaks at discotheques during which the ears can rest in a silent environment was increased. However, after the campaign, sound levels were more often judged as too loud, and the authors hypothesize that there might be less resistance for political action at that point.

It is possible that behavioural changes in adolescents are not achieved because the consequences of their behavior, hearing loss, is not immediately perceived or not experienced as serious enough. Widen and Erlandsson (2004) found that subjects reporting tinnitus and noise sensitivity are more worried regarding hearing loss than those without symptoms, and were more likely to report the use of hearing protectors [Widen and Erlandsson, 2004; Widen et al, 2006]. Moreover, subjects with permanent tinnitus assessed loud music-listening as more risky, and subjects with only occasional tinnitus listened more often to loud music [Bohlin and Erlandsson, 2007]. It was found that, even after perceiving hearing loss and/or tinnitus, only 14% was willing to avoid noisy leisure activities, 86% was prepared to reduce their attendance at such activities, and 12% did not have any intention to change their behavior regarding music exposure. So, previous hearing-related symptoms do not necessarily implicate a more responsible behavior in the future. However, they sometimes trigger behavioral changes [Bogoch et al, 2005].

The high sound levels in discotheques, concerts and parties are quite easily ascribed to the demands of the attendees by nightclub or discotheque owners and concert organizers. However, Mercier and Hohmann (2002) report that the sound levels are judged too high by 43%, 47% and 52% of the visitors in discotheques, concerts and techno parties, respectively. It was reported that the sound levels in discotheques was at least sometimes perceived as too loud by over 60% of adolescents [Weichbold and Zorowka, 2002], and it should be more quiet by more than 40% [Weichbold and Zorowka, 2005]. Also, at festivals, the sound levels were too loud for 25% of the attendees [Mercier et al, 2003]. It was even found that 85% of adolescents would not change their attendance behavior even if sound levels in discotheques were lowered, and almost 10% would visit discotheques more often when the sound levels were turned down [Weichbold and Zorowka, 2005]. Therefore, besides hearing conservation campaigns, more effort should be undertaken from politicians to regulate the sound levels in various establishments, as well as supervise the compliance of the legislation. Vogel et al (2008) also states that MP3 players should be equipped with a clear indicator of the volume, as well as with a warning signal when a hazardous doses is reached [Vogel et al, 2008].

Chapter 5

CASE STUDIES

1. SHORT-TERM AUDITORY EFFECTS

1.1. Case One

Case one represents a 26-year old male which participated at our current study on leisure noise exposure. He mentioned a five-hour attendance in a nightclub about nine hours before his visit. There was bilateral a normal otoscopy, type A tympanogram and present acoustic stapedial reflexes at 1.0 kHz. Pure-tone audiometry and DPOAEs were performed, and are reflected in Figure 1 and 2, respectively. Pure-tone audiometry revealed normal hearing at the right ear, and a audiometric notch of 30 dBHL at 4 kHz at the left ear. DPOAEs evoked with L1/L2=65/55 dBSPL showed reduced emission amplitudes at the right ear and significantly deteriorated amplitudes at the left ear.

1.2. Case Two

Case two is a 24-year old male participating at the study regarding the short-term auditory effects of listening to an MP3 player with supra-aural headphones during one hour. He listened to poprock music at a loud, but comfortable listening level. Pure-tone audiometry and DPOAEs (L1/L2=65/55 dBSPL) were measured before and after exposure. Normal otoscopy, type A tympanogram and normal acoustic stapedial reflexes at 1.0 kHz were obtained before music exposure. The results of the right ear for audiometry (Figure 3) and DPOAEs (Figure 4) are shown. Temporary thresholds shifts varied between 5 and 10 dB, which can be regarded as the test-retest reliability of hearing thresholds. The emission amplitudes decreased considerably; the largest temporary emissions shifts were 4.4, 6.1 and 4.0 dB at half-octave frequency band with centre frequencies 4.0, 6.0 and 8.0 kHz.

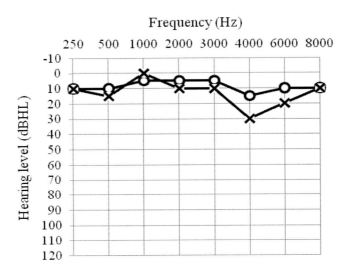

Figure 1. Hearing thresholds at octave frequencies from 250 to 8000 Hz, and half-octave frequencies 3000 and 6000 Hz for the right ear (circles) and left ear (crosses).

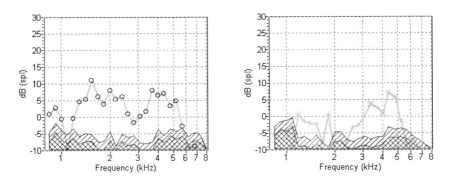

Figure 2. DPOAE amplitudes (grey lines) and noise amplitudes (shaded areas) from 841 to 8000 Hz for the right ear (right) and left ear (left).

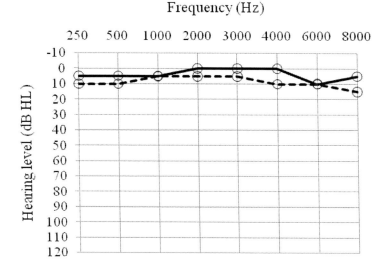

Figure 3. Pure-tone audiometry of case number two. The solid line represents the pre-exposure measurement; the dashed line the post-exposure measurement of listening to an MP3 player for one hour.

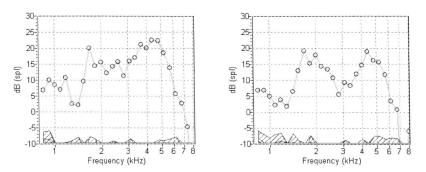

Figure 4. DPOAE amplitudes (grey lines) and noise amplitudes (shaded areas) of case two: pre-exposure measurement (right) and post-exposure measurement (left) of listening to an MP3 player for one hour.

2. LONG-TERM AUDITORY EFFECTS

2.1. Case Three

Case three is a 22-year-old male student participating at our current study regarding leisure noise exposure. There was a bilateral normal otoscopy, type A tympanogram and normal acoustic stapedial reflexes at 1.0 kHz. Pure-tone audiometry was measured (Figure 5) and shows bilateral (quasi-)normal hearing thresholds at conventional frequencies. Extended high-frequency audiometry was performed at 10.0, 12.5 and 16.0 kHz. Hearing thresholds were lowered, with the largest hearing loss of 60 dBHL at 16.0 kHz for the right ear. Figure 6 represents the DPOAEs (L1/L2=65/55 dBSPL) and reduced emission amplitudes are observed at both ears, with the left ear more deteriorated than the right ear. His noise exposure history can be described as substantially, as reflected in Table 1. He listens to his PMPs at maximum volume setting, mostly while using public transportation. After attending a discotheque, he usually experiences a post-exposure tinnitus.

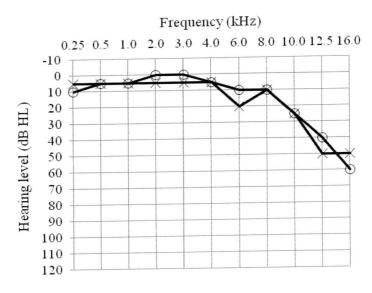

Figure 5. Reflected are the hearing thresholds at frequencies from 0.250 to 16.0 kHz of both ears (right ear: circles; left ear: crosses) of case number three.

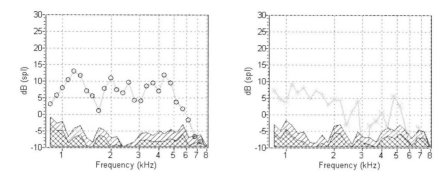

Figure 6. DPOAE amplitudes (grey lines) and noise amplitudes (shaded areas) for both ears (right ear: right; left ear: left) of case number three.

Table 1. Summary of the noise history of case number three

Leisure activity	Weekly or monthly exposure (hours)	Duration of exposure (years)
Listening to a PMP	9 hrs/wk	7
Listening to a stereo	14 hrs/wk	7
Attendance at discotheques or parties	15 hrs/wk	6
Attendance of live concerts	6 hrs/month	4
Visiting a cinema or theater	2 hrs/month	6
Attendance at sport events	5 hrs/wk	3

2.2. Case Four

Case four is a male of 22 years old. He also voluntarily participated at a current study regarding leisure noise exposure. Since six years, he experiences a hearing loss and tinnitus at both ears. A high-frequency hearing loss, especially at 4 and 6 kHz, was confirmed by a ENT-specialist. He wears hearing protector devices rigorously, and a hearing test is performed yearly. At the time of testing, normal otoscopy, type A tympanogram and normal acoustic stapedial reflexes at 1.0 kHz were obtained. Pure-tone audiometry (Figure 7) reveals bilateral high-frequency sensorineural hearing loss from 2.0 kHz at the left ear and 3.0 kHz at the right ear. DPOAEs (L1/L2=65/55 dBSPL) were measured and revealed absent emission amplitudes in the high-frequencies, and slightly more preserved emission amplitudes at the right ear (Figure 8).

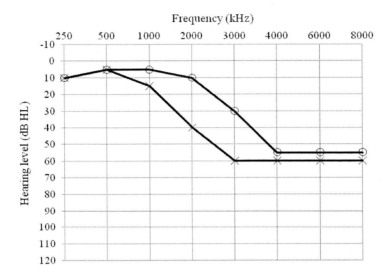

Figure 7. Pure-tone audiometry of case number four for the right ear (circles) and left ear (crosses).

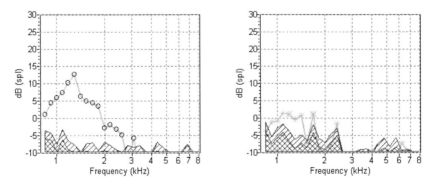

Figure 8. DPOAE amplitudes (grey lines) and noise amplitudes (shaded areas) measured in case number four for the right ear (right figure) and left ear (left figure).

3. CONCLUSION

These case studies illustrate the short- and long-term auditory effects of recreational noise exposure. In cases with hearing loss as established with pure-tone audiometry, the emission amplitudes are also reduced. Moreover, in cases with audiometric normal hearing, emission amplitudes indicate cochlear damage. Therefore, it can be concluded that OAEs complement pure-tone audiometry in the detection of cochlear hearing loss caused by noise exposure and more specifically leisure noise exposure. The clinical utility of OAEs in the diagnosis of (pre-clinical) NIHL must be further explored.

Chapter 6

REGULATION

There is increasing excessive noise exposure everywhere. Long-term exposure to high noise levels have caused moderate to severe hearing problems in millions of industrial workers [Dobie, 2008]. Moreover, recent studies of environmental noise have demonstrated that children compared to workers may receive more decibels from an 8-hour working day in a factory and that persons regularly attending sport events are exposed to intensity levels exceeding all federal guidelines (WHO, 1997).

Most of the guidelines, criteria and legislation are setup for occupational purposes. Estimations of the risk for developing a non-occupational hearing loss is nowadays compared to hearing loss caused by occupational exposure. The problem of noise and hearing conservation is regulated in specific standards, regulations and legislations for recordkeeping and the general industry. A regulation is a rule prescribed by the government and is more formal than a standard. A standard is a set of rules or guidelines, but can be developed also by consensus groups, such as the American National Standards Institute (ANSI). Legislation consists of laws prescribed by the American Congress or by local governing bodies [Sutter, 1996]. In Europe, these standards and legislations are expressed as European Community Directives. The most recent directive is Directive 2003-10-EC of the European Parliament and Council on the minimum health and safety requirements regarding the exposure of workers to the risks arising from physical agents (Directive 2003-10-EC, 2003). Other nations use a code of practice, which has less legal force than regulations and legislations. An example of this is the Australian national standard in which a 35 page code of practice provides the guidelines on how the standard, described in two short paragraphs, should be implemented.

Finally, recommendations are sometimes used, which act more as guidelines rather than enforceable rules [Sutter, 1996].

Most of these standards are based on little valid, reliable, and scientific data. Political, social and economical factors have often strong influence on the final rules and regulations. As a consequence permissible safety exposure limits (PEL), rules and guidelines differ very much according to country.

An overview of all standards, rules and regulations of the different countries and states is not within the scope of this chapter. As an example the different parameters of the 1910.95 OSHA Noise Standard are provided here (OSHA, 1992).

In the 1910.95 OSHA Noise Standard, PELs for noise are described as the maximum duration of exposure per working day, permitted for various noise intensity levels (in dBA). The exposure-duration table of the OSHA standard is described in Table 2.

Table 2. Permissible Noise Exposure (OSHA, 1992)

Exposure duration per day (hours)	Exposure level (dBA)
8	90
6	92
4	95
3	97
2	100
1	105
½	110
¼	115

The PELs depend on two parameters, a criterion level and an exchange rate. The criterion level is the steady noise intensity level, which is allowed for a full eight-hour working day. This is 90 dBA in most jurisdictions, but in Europe and other nations these values may be much lower.

Applying the equal-energy rule of sound, increasing the noise level above the criterion level, must result in a decrease of the allowed exposure time. This level-duration relation depends on the exchange rate. The exchange rate is the amount by which the permissible exposure level can be increased when the exposure duration is divided by two. There are worldwide two types of exchange rates in use: 3 dBA and 5 dBA exchange rates. These two exchange rates produce different guidelines worldwide. The 3 dBA exchange rate is more stringent. The maximum permitted duration for a 105 dBA noise exposure using the 3 dBA exchange rate is 15 minutes, whereas it is one hour with the 5 dBA exchange rate. Most international experts evaluate the 3 dBA rule as more logical for occupational noise exposure. As can be seen in Table 2, the OSHA advices a PEL of 90 dBA and an exchange rate of 5 dBA. The US Army and Air Force now use 3 dB exchange rates.

Since most of the regulations and standards across the world are made for occupational purposes, one should be cautious to extrapolate these criteria and permissible exposure levels to the situations of recreational noise exposure.

There is an increasing need for an international debate on legislation and regulation of noise exposure outside occupational activities. Legislation on output levels of PMPs and sound levels in discotheques, nightclubs, live concerts or at festivals is urgently needed and should not be based on occupational regulations and legislations.

Chapter 7

CONCLUSION

NIHL is the result of long-term noise exposure in the occupational setting, as well as during non-occupational, leisure activities. These leisure activities include participation in non-musical activities, as well as music-related exposure. The most common sources of music exposure during leisure activities are listening to PMPs, and attending discotheques, nightclubs, or live concerts.

An increased prevalence of NIHL in the youth caused by these leisure noise exposures is assumed in the mainstream media. However, scientific results concerning this issue are equivocal. There is a definite amount of high-frequency hearing loss in young people, but there are only small associations observed between recreational noise exposure and hearing loss as determined by pure-tone audiometry and clear, firm evidence of an increased prevalence of NIHL is not yet noticed.

Several explanations are possible. First, it could be that recreational noise exposure is insufficient to cause widespread hearing loss. Second, recent technological improvements in PMPs, and subsequently improved listening comfort and habits do not cause hearing loss yet. Finally, it is suggested that pure-tone audiometry is not sensitive enough to detect minimal cochlear damage.

Nevertheless, the aforementioned sources of leisure noise can be hazardous for hearing in some highly susceptible, or even in many young people with extreme listening or attendance habits. Therefore, further research on several domains is essentially to prevent NIHL in young people.

First, a careful inventory of leisure activities and listening habits in a representative sample of adolescents is needed, as well as a well-grounded understanding of music-listening habits. As mentioned above, there are gender differences in listening habits, and these habits also tend to change during life. Therefore, factors determining risk behavior regarding noise exposure must be further explored. We prefer a multidisciplinary context with at least a hearing specialist and psychologist to gain insight in risk behavior excessive music listening by adolescents.

Second, the long-term risk of cumulative noise exposures of adolescents must be evaluated. We recommend using OAEs and/or extended high-frequency audiometry complementary with conventional pure-tone audiometry. The usefulness of OAEs in the diagnosis of (pre-clinical) NIHL must be further explored, but are promising as indicated by our case studies.

Finally, hearing education campaigns should educate adolescents, and other parties involved in the prevention of NIHL. As education is not enough to induce behavioral changes in adolescents, we insist on a strict legislation to limit sound levels in several establishments with high intensity levels, as well as a limitation of the output levels of PMPs.

REFERENCES

Airo, E., Pekkarinen, J. and Olkinuora, P. S. (1996). Listening to music with earphones: an assessment of noise exposure. *Acta Acustica*, *82*, 885-94.

Alberti, P. (1998). Traumatic sensorineural hearing loss. In H. Ludman and A. Wright (Eds.), *Diseases of the ear* (6th, pp. 483-494). London: Arnold/Hodder Headline.

American College of Occupational and Environmental Medicine. (2002). Position Statement on noise-induced hearing loss. http://www.acoem.org/guidelines.

Arlinger, S. (2003). Negative consequences of uncorrected hearing loss--a review. *Int J Audiol*, *42 Suppl 2*, 2S17-20.

Attias, J., Horovitz, G., El-Hatib, N. and Nageris, B. (2001). Detection and Clinical Diagnosis of Noise-Induced Hearing Loss by Otoacoustic Emissions. *Noise Health*, *3*, 19-31.

Augustsson, I. and Engstrand, I. (2006). Hearing ability according to screening at conscription; comparison with earlier reports and with previous screening results for individuals without known ear disease. *Int J Pediatr Otorhinolaryngol*, *70*, 909-13.

Axelsson, A., Jerson, T., Lindberg, U. and Lindgren, F. (1981a). Early noise-induced hearing loss in teenage boys. *Scand Audiol*, *10*, 91-6.

Axelsson, A., Jerson, T. and Lindgren, F. (1981b). Noisy leisure time activities in teenage boys. *Am Ind Hyg Assoc J*, *42*, 229-33.

Axelsson, A. and Lindgren, F. (1978). Temporary threshold shift after exposure to pop music. *Scand Audiol*, *7*, 127-35.

Axelsson, A. and Prasher, D. (1999). Tinnitus: A warning signal to teenagers attending discotheques? *Noise Health*, *1*, 1-2.

Axelsson, A. and Prasher, D. (2000). Tinnitus induced by occupational and leisure noise. *Noise Health*, *2*, 47-54.

Axelsson, A., Rosenhall, U. and Zachau, G. (1994). Hearing in 18-year-old Swedish males. *Scand Audiol, 23*, 129-34.

Becher, S., Struwe, F., Schwenzer, C. and Weber, K. (1996). [Risk of hearing loss caused by high volume music--presenting an educational concept for preventing hearing loss in adolescents]. *Gesundheitswesen, 58*, 91-5.

Bhagat, S. P. and Davis, A. M. (2008). Modification of otoacoustic emissions following ear-level exposure to MP3 player music. *Int J Audiol, 47*, 751-60.

Biassoni, E. C. et al (2005). Recreational noise exposure and its effects on the hearing of adolescents. Part II: development of hearing disorders. *Int J Audiol, 44*, 74-85.

Bogoch, I. I., House, R. A. and Kudla, I. (2005). Perceptions about hearing protection and noise-induced hearing loss of attendees of rock concerts. *Can J Public Health, 96*, 69-72.

Bohlin, M. C. and Erlandsson, S. I. (2007). Risk behaviour and noise exposure among adolescents. *Noise Health, 9*, 55-63.

Bonfils, P., Bertrand, Y. and Uziel, A. (1988). Evoked otoacoustic emissions: normative data and presbycusis. *Audiology, 27*, 27-35.

Bradley, R., Fortnum, H. and Coles, R. (1987). Patterns of exposure of schoolchildren to amplified music. *Br J Audiol, 21*, 119-25.

Brownell, W. E. (1990). Outer hair cell electromotility and otoacoustic emissions. *Ear Hear, 11*, 82-92.

Carter, N. L., Murray, N., Khan, A. and Waugh, D. (1984). A longitudinal study of recreational noise and young people's hearing. *Australian Journal of Audiology, 6*, 45-53.

Carter, N. L., Waugh, R. L., Keen, K., Murray, N. and Bulteau, V. G. (1982). Amplified music and young people's hearing. Review and report of Australian findings. *Med J Aust, 2*, 125-8.

Catalano, P. J. and Levin, S. M. (1985). Noise-induced hearing loss and portable radios with headphones. *Int J Pediatr Otorhinolaryngol, 9*, 59-67.

Céranic, B. (2007). The value of otoacoustic emissions in the investigation of noise damage. *Audiological Medicine, 5*, 10-24.

Chung, J. H., Des Roches, C. M., Meunier, J. and Eavey, R. D. (2005). Evaluation of noise-induced hearing loss in young people using a web-based survey technique. *Pediatrics, 115*, 861-7.

Clark, W. W. (1991). Noise exposure from leisure activities: a review. *J Acoust Soc Am, 90*, 175-81.

Crandell, C., Mills, T. L. and Gauthier, R. (2004). Knowledge, behaviors, and attitudes about hearing loss and hearing protection among racial/ethnically diverse young adults. *J Natl Med Assoc*, *96*, 176-86.

Daniel, E. (2007). Noise and hearing loss: a review. *J Sch Health*, *77*, 225-31.

Davis, A. C., Lovell, E. A., Smith, P. A. and Ferguson, M. A. (1998). The contribution of social noise to tinnitus in young people - a preliminary report. *Noise Health*, *1*, 40-6.

Desai, A., Reed, D., Cheyne, A., Richards, S. and Prasher, D. (1999). Absence of otoacoustic emissions in subjects with normal audiometric thresholds implies exposure to noise. *Noise Health*, *1*, 58-65.

Dobie, R. A. (2008). The burdens of age-related and occupational noise-induced hearing loss in the United States. *Ear Hear*, *29*, 565-77.

European Parliament and Council. 2003. Directive 2003-10-EC on the minimum health and safety requirements regarding the exposure of workers to the risks arising from physical agents (noise), 2003-10-EC.

Fearn, R. W. and Hanson, D. R. (1984). Hearing damage in young people using headphone to listen to pop music. *Journal of sound and vibration*, *96*, 147-9.

Fligor, B. J. and Cox, L. C. (2004). Output levels of commercially available portable compact disc players and the potential risk to hearing. *Ear Hear*, *25*, 513-27.

Florentine, M., Hunter, W., Robinson, M., Ballou, M. and Buus, S. (1998). On the behavioral characteristics of loud-music listening. *Ear Hear*, *19*, 420-8.

Gissel, S., Mortensen, J. T. and Juul, S. (2002). Evaluation of hearing ability in Danish children at the time of school start and at the end of school. *Int J Adolesc Med Health*, *14*, 43-9.

Gorga, M. P. et al (1997). From laboratory to clinic: a large scale study of distortion product otoacoustic emissions in ears with normal hearing and ears with hearing loss. *Ear Hear*, *18*, 440-55.

Hall, A. J. and Lutman, M. E. (1999). Methods for early identification of noise-induced hearing loss. *Audiology*, *38*, 277-80.

Hanson, D. R. and Fearn, R. W. (1975). Hearing acuity in young people exposed to pop music and other noise. *Lancet*, *2*, 203-5.

Hausler, R. (2004). [The effects of acoustic overstimulation]. *Ther Umsch*, *61*, 21-9.

Heinrich, U. and Feltens, R. (2006). Mechanisms underlying noise-induced hearing loss. *Drug Discovery Today: Disease Mechanisms*, *3*, 131-5.

Hellstrom, P. A. (1991). The effects on hearing from portable cassette players: a follow-up study. *Journal of sound and vibration, 151*, 461-9.

Hellstrom, P. A., Axelsson, A. and Costa, O. (1998). Temporary threshold shift induced by music. *Scand Audiol Suppl, 48*, 87-94.

Henderson, D., Bielefeld, E. C., Harris, K. C. and Hu, B. H. (2006). The role of oxidative stress in noise-induced hearing loss. *Ear Hear, 27*, 1-19.

Henderson, D., Subramaniam, M. and Boettcher, F. A. (1993). Individual susceptibility to noise-induced hearing loss: an old topic revisited. *Ear Hear, 14*, 152-68.

Hetu, R. and Fortin, M. (1995). Potential risk of hearing damage associated with exposure to highly amplified music. *J Am Acad Audiol, 6*, 378-86.

Hodgetts, W. E., Rieger, J. M. and Szarko, R. A. (2007). The effects of listening environment and earphone style on preferred listening levels of normal hearing adults using an MP3 player. *Ear Hear, 28*, 290-7.

Holmes, A. E., Niskar, A. S., Kieszak, S. M., Rubin, C. and Brody, D. J. (2004). Mean and median hearing thresholds among children 6 to 19 years of age: the Third National Health And Nutrition Examination Survey, 1988 to 1994, United States. *Ear Hear, 25*, 397-402.

Hotz, M. A., Probst, R., Harris, F. P. and Hauser, R. (1993). Monitoring the effects of noise exposure using transiently evoked otoacoustic emissions. *Acta Otolaryngol, 113*, 478-82.

Hu, B. H., Henderson, D. and Nicotera, T. M. (2002). Involvement of apoptosis in progression of cochlear lesion following exposure to intense noise. *Hear Res, 166*, 62-71.

Ising, H. (1994). [Potential hearing loss caused by loud music. Current status of knowledge and need for management]. *HNO, 42*, 465-6.

Ising, H., Babisch, W., Hanel, J., Kruppa, B. and Pilgramm, M. (1995). [Empirical studies of music listening habits of adolescents. Optimizing sound threshold limits for cassette players and discoteques]. *HNO, 43*, 244-9.

Ising, H., Hanel, J., Pilgramm, M., Babisch, W. and Lindthammer, A. (1994). [Risk of hearing loss caused by listening to music with head phones]. *HNO, 42*, 764-8.

Jokitulppo, J. and Bjork, E. (2002). Estimated leisure-time noise exposure and hearing symptoms in a finnish urban adult population. *Noise Health, 5*, 53-62.

Jokitulppo, J., Toivonen, M. and Bjork, E. (2006). Estimated leisure-time noise exposure, hearing thresholds, and hearing symptoms of Finnish conscripts. *Mil Med, 171*, 112-6.

Jokitulppo, J. S., Bjork, E. A. and kaan-Penttila, E. (1997). Estimated leisure noise exposure and hearing symptoms in Finnish teenagers. *Scand Audiol*, *26*, 257-62.

Keith, S. E., Michaud, D. S. and Chiu, V. (2008). Evaluating the maximum playback sound levels from portable digital audio players. *J Acoust Soc Am*, *123*, 4227-37.

Kemp, D. T. (1978). Stimulated acoustic emissions from within the human auditory system. *J Acoust Soc Am*, *64*, 1386-91.

Konopka, W., Zalewski, P. and Pietkiewicz, P. (2001). Evaluation of Transient and Distortion Product Otoacoustic Emissions before and after shooting practice. *Noise Health*, *3*, 29-37.

Kowalska, S. and Sulkowski, W. (1997). Measurements of click-evoked otoacoustic emission in industrial workers with noise-induced hearing loss. *Int J Occup Med Environ Health*, *10*, 441-59.

Lapsley-Miller, J.A., Marshall, L. and Heller, L.M. (2004). A longitudinal study of changes in evoked otoacoustic emissions and pure-tone thresholds as measured in a hearing conservation program. *Int J Audiol*, *43*, 307-22.

Le Prell, C. G., Yamashita, D., Minami, S. B., Yamasoba, T. and Miller, J. M. (2007). Mechanisms of noise-induced hearing loss indicate multiple methods of prevention. *Hear Res*, *226*, 22-43.

Lee, P. C., Senders, C. W., Gantz, B. J. and Otto, S. R. (1985). Transient sensorineural hearing loss after overuse of portable headphone cassette radios. *Otolaryngol Head Neck Surg*, *93*, 622-5.

Lees, R. E., Roberts, J. H. and Wald, Z. (1985). Noise induced hearing loss and leisure activities of young people: a pilot study. *Can J Public Health*, *76*, 171-3.

LePage, E. L. (1998). Occupational noise-induced hearing loss: origin, characterisation and prevention. *Acoustics Australia*, *26*, 57-61.

LePage, E. L. and Murray, N. M. (1998). Latent cochlear damage in personal stereo users: a study based on click-evoked otoacoustic emissions. *Med J Aust*, *169*, 588-92.

Liebel, J., Delb, W., Andes, C. and Koch, A. (1996). [Detection of hearing loss in patrons of a discoteque using TEOAE and DPOAE]. *Laryngorhinootologie*, *75*, 259-64.

Lindeman, H. E., van der Klaauw, M. M. and Platenburg-Gits, F. A. (1987). Hearing acuity in male adolescents (young adults) at the age of 17 to 23 years. *Audiology*, *26*, 65-78.

Lindgren, F. and Axelsson, A. (1983). Temporary threshold shift after exposure to noise and music of equal energy. *Ear Hear*, *4*, 197-201.

Lipscomb, D. M. (1972). The increase in prevalence of high frequency hearing impairment among college students. *Audiology*, *11*, 231-7.

Litke, R. E. (1971). Elevated high-frequency hearing in school children. *Arch Otolaryngol*, *94*, 255-7.

Loth, D., Avan, P., Menguy, C. and Teyssou, M. (1992). [Secondary auditory risks from listening to portable digital compact disc players]. *Bull Acad Natl Med*, *176*, 1245-52.

Lucertini, M., Moleti, A. and Sisto, R. (2002). On the detection of early cochlear damage by otoacoustic emission analysis. *J Acoust Soc Am*, *111*, 972-8.

Maassen, M. et al (2001). Ear damage caused by leisure noise. *Noise Health*, *4*, 1-16.

MacLean, G. L., Stuart, A. and Stenstrom, R. (1992). Real ears sound pressure levels developed by three portable stereo system earphones. *Am J Audiol* 52-5.

Mansfield, J. D., Baghurst, P. A. and Newton, V. E. (1999). Otoacoustic emissions in 28 young adults exposed to amplified music. *Br J Audiol*, *33*, 211-22.

Meecham, E. A. and Hume, K. I. (2001). Tinnitus, attendance at night-clubs and social drug taking in students. *Noise Health*, *3*, 53-62.

Melnick, W. (1991). Human temporary threshold shift (TTS) and damage risk. *J Acoust Soc Am*, *90*, 147-54.

Mercier, V. and Hohmann, B. W. (2002). Is Electronically Amplified Music too Loud? What do Young People Think? *Noise Health*, *4*, 47-55.

Mercier, V., Luy, D. and Hohmann, B. W. (2003). The sound exposure of the audience at a music festival. *Noise Health*, *5*, 51-8.

Metternich, F. U. and Brusis, T. (1999). [Acute hearing loss and tinnitus caused by amplified recreational music]. *Laryngorhinootologie*, *78*, 614-9.

Meyer-Bisch, C. (1996). Epidemiological evaluation of hearing damage related to strongly amplified music (personal cassette players, discotheques, rock concerts)--high-definition audiometric survey on 1364 subjects. *Audiology*, *35*, 121-42.

Mills, J. H. and Going, J. A. (1982). Review of environmental factors affecting hearing. *Environ Health Perspect*, *44*, 119-27.

Montgomery, J. K. and Fujikawa, S. (1992). Hearing thresholds of students in the second, eighth, and twelfth grades. *Language, Speech, and Hearing Services in School*, *23*, 61-3.

Montoya, F. S., Ibarguen, A. M., Vences, A. R., del Rey, A. S. and Fernandez, J. M. (2008). Evaluation of cochlear function in normal-hearing young adults exposed to MP3 player noise by analyzing transient evoked otoacoustic emissions and distortion products. *J Otolaryngol Head Neck Surg, 37,* 718-24.

Morata, T. C. (2007). Young people: their noise and music exposures and the risk of hearing loss. *Int J Audiol, 46,* 111-2.

Mostafapour, S. P., Lahargoue, K. and Gates, G. A. (1998). Noise-induced hearing loss in young adults: the role of personal listening devices and other sources of leisure noise. *Laryngoscope, 108,* 1832-9.

MRC Institute of Hearing Research (1986). Damage to hearing arising from leisure noise. *Br J Audiol, 20,* 157-64.

Niskar, A. S. et al (1998). Prevalence of hearing loss among children 6 to 19 years of age: the Third National Health and Nutrition Examination Survey. *JAMA, 279,* 1071-5.

Niskar, A. S. et al (2001). Estimated prevalence of noise-induced hearing threshold shifts among children 6 to 19 years of age: the Third National Health and Nutrition Examination Survey, 1988-1994, United States. *Pediatrics, 108,* 40-3.

Nordmann, A. S., Bohne, B. A. and Harding, G. W. (2000). Histopathological differences between temporary and permanent threshold shift. *Hear Res, 139,* 13-30.

Norton, S. J. (1992). Cochlear function and otoacoustic emissions. *Seminars in Hearing, 13,* 1-14.

Occupational Safety and Health Administration. 1992. Occupational Noise Exposure, 1910-95.

Opperman, D. A., Reifman, W., Schlauch, R. and Levine, S. (2006). Incidence of spontaneous hearing threshold shifts during modern concert performances. *Otolaryngol Head Neck Surg, 134,* 667-73.

Passchier-Vermeer, W. (1999). Pop music trough headphones and hearing loss. *Noise Control Eng J, 47,* 182-6.

Peng, J. H., Tao, Z. Z. and Huang, Z. W. (2007). Risk of damage to hearing from personal listening devices in young adults. *J Otolaryngol, 36,* 181-5.

Persson, B. O., Svedberg, A. and Gothe, C. J. (1993). Longitudinal changes in hearing ability among Swedish conscripts. *Scand Audiol, 22,* 141-3.

Plath, P. (1998a). [Socio-acousis. Non-occupationally-induced hearing loss due to noise, 1]. *HNO, 46,* 887-92.

Plath, P. (1998b). [Sociacusis. Non-occupationally induced hearing damage by noise, 2]. *HNO, 46,* 947-52.

Plinkert, P.K., Hemmert, W. and Zenner, H.P. (1995). [Comparison of methods for early detection of noise vulnerability of the inner ear. Amplitude reduction of otoacoustic emissions are most sensitive at submaximal noise impulse exposure]. *HNO, 43*, 89-97.

Probst, R., Lonsbury-Martin, B. L. and Martin, G. K. (1991). A review of otoacoustic emissions. *J Acoust Soc Am, 89*, 2027-67.

Probst, R., Harris, F.P. and Hauser, R. (1993). Clinical monitoring using otoacoustic emissions. *Br J Audiol, 27*, 85-90.

Pugsley, S., Stuart, A., Kalinowski, J. and Armson, J. (1993). Changes in hearing sensitivity following portable stereo system use. *Am J Audiol, 2*, 64-7.

Rabinowitz, P. M., Slade, M. D., Galusha, D., xon-Ernst, C. and Cullen, M. R. (2006). Trends in the prevalence of hearing loss among young adults entering an industrial workforce 1985 to 2004. *Ear Hear, 27*, 369-75.

Rawool, V. W. and Colligon-Wayne, L. A. (2008). Auditory lifestyles and beliefs related to hearing loss among college students in the USA. *Noise Health, 10*, 1-10.

Rice, C. G., Rossi, G. and Olina, M. (1987a). Damage risk from personal cassette players. *Br J Audiol, 21*, 279-88.

Rice, C.G., Breslin, M. and Roper, R.G. (1987b). Sound levels from personal cassette players. *Br J Audiol, 21*, 273-278.

Schmuziger, N., Fostiropoulos, K. and Probst, R. (2006). Long-term assessment of auditory changes resulting from a single noise exposure associated with non-occupational activities. *Int J Audiol, 45*, 46-54.

Serra, M. R. et al (2005). Recreational noise exposure and its effects on the hearing of adolescents. Part I: an interdisciplinary long-term study. *Int J Audiol, 44*, 65-73.

Shah, S., Gopal, B., Reis, J. and Novak, M. (2009). Hear today, gone tomorrow: an assessment of portable entertainment player use and hearing acuity in a community sample. *J Am Board Fam Med, 22*, 17-23.

Sliwinska-Kowalska, M. and Jedlinska, U. (1998). Prolonged exposure to industrial noise: cochlear pathology does not correlate with the degree of permanent threshold shift, but is related to duration of exposure. *J Occup Health, 40*, 123-31.

Sliwinska-Kowalska, M. and Kotylo, P. (2007). Evaluation of individuals with known or suspected noise damage to hearing. *Audiological Medicine, 5*, 54-65.

Smith, P. A., Davis, A., Ferguson, M. and Lutman, M. E. (2000). The prevalence and type of social noise exposure in young adults in England. *Noise Health, 2*, 41-56.

Spaeth, J., Klimek, L., Doring, W. H., Rosendahl, A. and Mosges, R. (1993). [How badly does the "normal-hearing" young man of 1992 hear in the high frequency range?]. *HNO, 41*, 385-8.

Strauss, P., Quante, M., Strahl, M., Averhage, H. and Bitzer, M. (1977). [Is hearing of the students damaged by environmental noise in their leisure time?]. *Laryngol Rhinol Otol (Stuttg), 56*, 868-71.

Sutter, A. H. (1996). Current Standards for Occupational Exposure to Noise. In A. Axelsson et al. (Eds.), *Scientific Basis of Noise-Induced Hearing Loss*New York: Thieme Medical Publishers.

Swanson, S. J., Dengerink, H. A., Kondrick, P. and Miller, C. L. (1987). The influence of subjective factors on temporary threshold shifts after exposure to music and noise of equal energy. *Ear Hear, 8*, 288-91.

Talaska, A. E. and Schacht, J. (2007). Mechanisms of noise damage to the cochlea. *Audiological Medicine, 5*, 3-9.

Torre, P., III (2008). Young adults' use and output level settings of personal music systems. *Ear Hear, 29*, 791-9.

Turunen-Rise, I., Flottorp, G. and Tvete, O. (1991). Personal cassette players ('Walkman'). Do they cause noise-induced hearing loss? *Scand Audiol, 20*, 239-44.

Vogel, I., Brug, J., Hosli, E. J., van der Ploeg, C. P. and Raat, H. (2008). MP3 players and hearing loss: adolescents' perceptions of loud music and hearing conservation. *J Pediatr, 152*, 400-4.

Vogel, I., Brug, J., van der Ploeg, C. P. and Raat, H. (2009a). Prevention of adolescents' music-induced hearing loss due to discotheque attendance: a Delphi study. *Health Educ Res*.

Vogel, I., Brug, J., van der Ploeg, C. P. and Raat, H. (2009b). Strategies for the prevention of MP3-induced hearing loss among adolescents: expert opinions from a Delphi study. *Pediatrics, 123*, 1257-62.

Vogel, I., Brug, J., van der Ploeg, C. P. and Raat, H. (2007). Young people's exposure to loud music: a summary of the literature. *Am J Prev Med, 33*, 124-33.

Weichbold, V. and Zorowka, P. (2002). [Effect of information about hearing damage caused by loud music. For adolescents the music in discoteques is too loud despite loudness limits]. *HNO, 50*, 560-4.

Weichbold, V. and Zorowka, P. (2005). [Will adolescents visit discotheque less often if sound levels of music are decreased?]. *HNO, 53*, 845-1.

Weichbold, V. and Zorowka, P. (2007). Can a hearing education campaign for adolescents change their music listening behavior? *Int J Audiol, 46,* 128-33.

Weichbold, V. and Zorowka, P. (2003). Effects of a hearing protection campaign on the discotheque attendance habits of high-school students. *Int J Audiol, 42,* 489-93.

West, P. D. and Evans, E. F. (1990). Early detection of hearing damage in young listeners resulting from exposure to amplified music. *Br J Audiol, 24,* 89-103.

Widen, S. E. and Erlandsson, S. I. (2004). Self-reported tinnitus and noise sensitivity among adolescents in Sweden. *Noise Health, 7,* 29-40.

Widen, S. E., Holmes, A. E. and Erlandsson, S. I. (2006). Reported hearing protection use in young adults from Sweden and the USA: effects of attitude and gender. *Int J Audiol, 45,* 273-80.

Williams, W. (2005). Noise exposure levels from personal stereo use. *Int J Audiol, 44,* 231-6.

Wong, T. W., Van Hasselt, C. A., Tang, L. S. and Yiu, P. C. (1990). The use of personal cassette players among youths and its effects on hearing. *Public Health, 104,* 327-30.

World Health Organization. 1997. Prevention of noise-induced hearing loss: report of an informal consultation held at the World Health Organization, Geneva, on 28-30 October 1997.

Yassi, A., Pollock, N., Tran, N. and Cheang, M. (1993). Risks to hearing from a rock concert. *Can Fam Physician, 39,* 1045-50.

Zenner, H. P. et al (1999). [Hearing loss caused by leisure noise]. *HNO, 47,* 236-48.

Zogby, J. (2006). Survey of teens and adults about the use of personal electronic devices and head phones. *Am Speech Lang Hear Assoc.*

INDEX